TABLE OF CONTENTS

INTRODUCTION

Cervical cancer begins when healthy cells on the surface of the cervix change and grow out of control, forming a mass called a tumor. A tumor can be cancerous or benign. A cancerous tumor is malignant, meaning it can spread to other parts of the body. A benign tumor means the tumor will not spread.

At first, the changes in a cell are abnormal, not cancerous. Researchers believe that some of these abnormal changes are the first step in a series of slow changes that can lead to cancer. Some of the abnormal cells go away without treatment, but others can become cancerous. This phase of the disease is called dysplasia, which is an abnormal growth of cells. The abnormal cells, sometimes called precancerous tissue, need to be removed to stop cancer from developing. Often, the precancerous tissue can be removed or destroyed without harming healthy tissue, but in some cases, a hysterectomy is needed to prevent cervical cancer. A hysterectomy is the removal of the uterus and cervix.

Cervical cancer is a type of cancer that starts in the cervix. The cervix is a hollow cylinder that connects the lower part of a woman's uterus to her vagina. Most cervical cancers begin in cells on the surface of the cervix.

SYMPTOMS OF CERVICAL CANCER

Many women with cervical cancer don't realize they have the disease early on, because it usually doesn't cause symptoms until the late stages. When symptoms do appear, they're easily mistaken for common conditions like menstrual periods and urinary tract infections (UTIs).

Typical cervical cancer symptoms are:

unusual bleeding, such as in between periods, after sex, or after menopause

vaginal discharge that looks or smells different than usual

pain in the pelvis

needing to urinate more often

pain during urination

If you notice any of these symptoms, see your doctor for an exam. Find out how your doctor will diagnose cervical cancer.

CERVICAL CANCER CAUSES

Most cervical cancer cases are caused by the sexually transmitted human papillomavirus (HPV). This is the same virus that causes genital warts.

There are about 100 different strains of HPV. Only certain types cause cervical cancer. The two types that most commonly cause cancer are HPV-16 and HPV-18.

Being infected with a cancer-causing strain of HPV doesn't mean you'll get cervical cancer. Your immune system eliminates the vast majority of HPV infections, often within two years.

HPV can also cause other cancers in women and men. These include:

vulvar cancer

vaginal cancer

penile cancer

anal cancer

rectal cancer

ALEX PAUL M.D

throat cancer

HPV is a very common infection. Find out what percentage of sexually active adults will get it at some point in their lifetime.

CERVICAL CANCER TREATMENT

Cervical cancer is very treatable if you catch it early. The four main treatments are:

surgery

radiation therapy

chemotherapy

targeted therapy

Sometimes these treatments are combined to make them more effective.

Surgery

The purpose of surgery is to remove as much of the cancer as possible. Sometimes the doctor can remove just the area of the cervix that contains cancer cells. For cancer that's more widespread, surgery may involve removing the cervix and other organs in the pelvis.

Radiation therapy

Radiation kills cancer cells using high-energy X-ray beams. It can be delivered through a machine outside the body. It can also be delivered from inside the body using a metal tube placed in the uterus or vagina.

Chemotherapy

Chemotherapy uses drugs to kill cancer cells throughout the body. Doctors give this treatment in cycles. You'll get chemo for a period of time. You'll then stop the treatment to give your body time to recover.

Targeted therapy

Bevacizumab (Avastin) is a newer drug that works in a different way from chemotherapy and radiation. It blocks the growth of new blood vessels that help the cancer grow and survive. This drug is often given together with chemotherapy.

If your doctor discovers precancerous cells in your cervix they can be treated. See what methods stop these cells from turning into cancer.

CERVICAL CANCER STAGES

After you've been diagnosed, your doctor will assign your cancer a stage. The stage tells whether the cancer has spread, and if so, how far it's spread. Staging your cancer can help your doctor find the right treatment for you.

Cervical cancer has four stages:

Stage 1: The cancer is small. It may have spread to the lymph nodes. It hasn't spread to other parts of your body.

Stage 2: The cancer is larger. It may have spread outside of the uterus and cervix or to the lymph nodes. It still hasn't reached other parts of your body.

Stage 3: The cancer has spread to the lower part of the vagina or to the pelvis. It may be blocking the ureters, the tubes that carry urine from the kidneys to the bladder. It hasn't spread to other parts of your body.

Stage 4: The cancer may have spread outside of the pelvis to organs like your lungs, bones, or liver.

Cervical cancer test

A Pap smear is a test doctors use to diagnose cervical cancer. To perform this test, your doctor collects a sample of cells from the surface of your cervix. These cells are then sent to a lab to be tested for precancerous or cancerous changes.

If these changes are found, your doctor may suggest a colposcopy, a procedure for examining your cervix. During this test, your doctor might take a biopsy, which is a sample of cervical cells.

Ages 21 to 29: Get a Pap smear once every three years.

Ages 30 to 65: Get a Pap smear once every three years, get a high-risk HPV (hrHPV) test every five years, or get a Pap smear plus hrHPV test every five years.

CERVICAL CANCER RISK FACTORS

HPV is the biggest risk for cervical cancer. Other factors that can also increase your risk include:

human immunodeficiency virus (HIV)

chlamydia

smoking

obesity

a family history of cervical cancer

a diet low in fruits and vegetables

taking birth control pills

having three full-term pregnancies

being younger than 17 when you got pregnant for the first time

Even if you have one or more of these factors, you're not destined to get cervical cancer

Cervical cancer prognosis

For cervical cancer that's caught in the early stages, when it's still confined to the cervix, the five-year survival rate is 92 percent.

Once the cancer has spread within the pelvic area, the five-year survival rate drops to 56 percent. If the cancer spreads to distant parts of the body, survival is just 17 percent.

Routine testing is important for improving the outlook of women with cervical cancer. When this cancer is caught early, it's very treatable.

CERVICAL CANCER SURGERY

Several different types of surgery treat cervical cancer. Which one your doctor recommends depends on how far the cancer has spread.

Cryosurgery freezes cancer cells with a probe placed in the cervix.

Laser surgery burns off abnormal cells with a laser beam.

Conization removes a cone-shaped section of the cervix using a surgical knife, laser, or a thin wire heated by electricity.

Hysterectomy removes the entire uterus and cervix. When the top of the vagina is also removed, it's called a radical hysterectomy.

Trachelectomy removes the cervix and the top of the vagina, but leaves the uterus in place so that a woman can have children in the future.

Pelvic exenteration may remove the uterus, vagina, bladder, rectum, lymph nodes, and part of the colon, depending on where the cancer has spread.

Cervical cancer prevention

One of the easiest ways to prevent cervical cancer is by getting screened regularly with a Pap smear and/or hrHPV test. Screening picks up precancerous cells, so they can be treated before they turn into cancer.

HPV infection causes most cervical cancer cases. The infection is preventable with the vaccines Gardasil and Cervarix. Vaccination is most effective before a person becomes sexually active. Both boys and girls can be vaccinated against HPV.

Here are a few other ways you can reduce your risk of HPV and cervical cancer:

limit the number of sexual partners you have

always use a condom or other barrier method when you have vaginal, oral, or anal sex

An abnormal Pap smear result indicates you have precancerous cells in your cervix. Find out what to do if your test comes back positive.

CERVICAL CANCER STATISTICS

Here are some key statistics about cervical cancer.

The American Cancer Society estimates that in 2019, approximately 13,170 American women will be diagnosed with cervical cancer and 4,250 will die from the disease. Most cases will be diagnosed in women between the ages of 35 and 44.

Hispanic women are the most likely ethnic group to get cervical cancer in the United States. American Indians and Alaskan natives have the lowest rates.

The death rate from cervical cancer has dropped over the years. From 2002-2016, the number of deaths was 2.3 per 100,000 women per year. In part, this decline was due to improved screening.

Cervical cancer and pregnancy

It's rare to get diagnosed with cervical cancer while you're pregnant, but it can happen. Most cancers found during pregnancy are discovered at an early stage.

Treating cancer while you're pregnant can be complicated. Your doctor can help you decide on a treatment based on the stage of your cancer and how far along you're in your pregnancy.

If the cancer is at a very early stage, you may be able to wait to deliver before starting treatment. For a case of more advanced cancer where treatment requires a hysterectomy or radiation, you'll need to decide whether to continue the pregnancy.

FIGHTING CERVICAL CANCER WITH DIET

"Lots of research points to great benefits associated with diet and cancer. Eating mostly a plant-based diet — one that is made up primarily of fruits, vegetables, beans and whole grains — is the best

You can find ways to include these foods in your diet throughout the day. Moores recommends adding a variety of colors to your diet and including nutritious foods with attributes that fight cervical cancer at all three meals. For example:

Breakfast: orange juice, cantaloupe, yogurt, and granola

Lunch: open-faced toasted cheese and veggie sandwich with red peppers, carrots, mushrooms, and zucchini

Dinner: tossed romaine salad with grapefruit segments and whole-wheat pasta with spinach, black beans, chicken, and diced tomatoes

Flavonoids to Reduce Cervical Cancer Risk

Flavonoids are chemical compounds in fruits and vegetables that are thought to be a leading source protection against cancer. The following are just a few examples of flavonoid-rich foods to consider adding to your diet:

Apples

Asparagus

Black beans

Broccoli

Brussels sprouts

Cabbage

Cranberries

Garlic

Lettuce

Lima beans

Onions

Soy

Spinach

Folate as a Cervical Cancer Risk Reducer

Studies suggest that foods rich in folate (a water-soluble B vitamin) reduce the risk of cervical cancer in people with HPV. However, researchers do not yet know how folate might affect cancer risk. It is possible that folate helps the body stop HPV infection from coming back repeatedly, which decreases the risk of developing cancer.

Foods rich in folate include:

Avocados

Chickpeas

Fortified cereals and breads

Lentils

Orange juice

Romaine lettuce

Strawberries

Carotenoids in the Cervical Cancer Diet

Some studies suggest that carotenoids, a source of vitamin A, are also helpful in preventing cervical cancer risk. In addition to the fruits, vegetables, and beans on the lists above, you could also include orange foods such as carrots, sweet potatoes, pumpkin, and winter squash in your diet.

Cervical Cancer: Diet Is Only Part of the Solution

However, a diet high in fruits and vegetables — although an important part of an overall cancer prevention plan — cannot prevent cervical cancer by itself.

A healthy lifestyle that can help reduce your chances of developing cervical cancer should also include:

Getting annual Pap smears to screen for early cell changes

Getting vaccinated against HPV

Not smoking

Being monogamous (the risk of HPV increases with more than one sex partner)

Taking these steps and eating a diet high in fruits and

vegetables can help you keep your cervical cancer risk low

FOODS THAT FIGHT CERVICAL CANCER

Sweet Potatoes

Many yellow and orange fruits and vegetables contain beta-carotene. This antioxidant can prevent and treat several variations of cancer, including cervical. Sweet potatoes are one of the greatest sources of beta-carotene that are worth adding to your diet. They are much healthier than regular potatoes and can be enjoyed baked or mashed. It's important to consume the outer skin portion as well. Many of the nutrients are found there.

Spinach

Dark leafy greens offer folic acid. Folic acid helps in the building of new cells. These new cells can help to push out the damaged, toxic cells that are causing the cervical cancer and other diseases within the body. Spinach is an ideal source of other vitamins as well, such as Vitamin E. This vitamin works toward improving healthy cell function.

Carrots

Carrots contain lots of nutrients that aid in the fight against diseases. The antioxidants found in this vegetable are especially helpful in the battle against cervical cancer because they target the human papilloma virus. HPV is a common cause of cervical cancer. Having a diet rich in foods that target this disease is a major hep.

Apples

Apples provide a hefty dose of Vitamin C, which acts as an antioxidant that can fight off disease within the body. Many people up their Vitamin C intake when they have a common cold, not realizing that the nutritional value from it can help other ailments as well, including cervical cancer. An apple a day keeping the doctor away is a valid saying because of this.

Eggs

Protein is necessary to heal the body and repair damaged tissues. Eggs are an excellent source of protein, making them vital to eat during a battle with cancer of any kind. Lean meats and low-fat dairy products, such as yogurt, are also vital.

Cervical cancer, or any form of cancer for that matter, can be fought. A healthy diet is going to work wonders in combating symptoms and reducing the size of the toxic cells within the body. Combine this with exercise, regular check-ups with a doctor, and even chiropractic care that can help reduce stress levels and boost the immune system, and you are on the right track toward improving overall well-being.

RECIPES FOR CERVICAL CANCER

Asparagus with Quince Jam and Walnuts

Ingredients

2 lbs asparagus spears, washed and trimmed

2 tsp fresh ginger, grated

2 tbsp quince jam

2 tbsp extra-virgin olive oil

1 tsp lemon juice

3 tbsp walnuts, chopped

Salt and freshly ground black pepper, to taste

Directions

Prepare a steamer with boiling water. Add asparagus, cover, and steam until tender crisp, about 3-5 minutes. Transfer hot asparagus to a serving plate.

In a small bowl, whisk together ginger, quince jam, olive oil, lemon juice, and salt and pepper. Pour over asparagus. Sprinkle with chopped walnuts.

GRANDMA'S CHICKEN SOUP

Ingredients

4 cups fat-free, low-sodium chicken broth

1 onion, chopped

3/4 cup sweet potato, diced

3/4 cup turnip, diced

2 ribs organic celery, diced

2 carrots, sliced

1/2 cup fresh parsley, chopped

2 cups skinless, organic chicken, cooked and diced

Directions

Bring broth to a boil in a large saucepan, and add vegetables. Reduce heat to low, cover and simmer, until vegetables are tender.

Add cooked chicken and simmer for 3-4 minutes.

Super-Nutritious Broccoli Salad with Apples and Cranberries

This low-GI broccoli salad featuring apples and cranberries is low in calories and low in fat, but loaded with a wide range of nutrients.

RECIPE FOR BROCCOLI SALAD WITH APPLES AND CRANBERRIES

Ingredients

4 cups fresh broccoli florets

1/2 cup dried cranberries

1/2 cup sunflower seeds

3 organic apples

1/4 cup red onion, chopped

1 cup plain, low-fat yoghurt with probiotic bacteria

2 Tbsp Dijon style mustard

1/4 cup honey

Directions

Combine broccoli florets, dried cranberries, sunflower seeds, chopped apples, and chopped onion in a large serving bowl. Blend yoghurt, mustard, and honey in a small bowl.

Add dressing to the salad and toss. Chill before serving.

Red Cabbage Soup with Black Lentils

Ingredients

½ cup (96 g) black lentils

2 Tbsp (30 ml) olive oil

2 cloves (6 g) garlic

1 small onion (70 g)

½ red cabbage (420 g), shredded

2 ½ US cups (591 ml) low-sodium vegetable stock

½ broccoli (304 g), coarsely chopped

10 sprigs (5 g) fresh thyme, chopped

Directions

Prepare and cook the lentils according to the instructions on the package. While the lentils are cooking, chop the garlic and onions, and let them sit for 15 minutes to allow them to produce allicin, a health promoting compound that is formed when Allium vegetables such as garlic and onions are chopped.

Heat the olive oil in a large pan and add the garlic, onion, and red cabbage. Cook for a few minutes.

Add the vegetable stock and bring to a boil, then add the broccoli. Reduce heat, and simmer until the broccoli is tender. This generally takes about 8-10 minutes. Turn off the heat and stir in the cooked lentils. Add the thyme and serve immediately.

ROMAINE AND SMOKED SALMON SALAD

Ingredients

1 small head organic romaine lettuce

5 ounces smoked salmon, thinly sliced

2 tomatoes, diced

4 radishes, thinly sliced

1 organic carrot, diagonally sliced

1/2 cucumber, peeled and diced

Juice of half a lemon

1 tsp fresh ginger root, peeled and minced

1 tbsp canola oil

Directions

Arrange romaine lettuce on two plates. Top with salmon, tomatoes, radishes, carrots, and cucumber.

Shake lemon juice, canola oil, and minced ginger in tightly

covered jar. Pour over salad

Tomato, Cucumber and Red Onion Salad

Ingredients

2 large cucumbers, peeled and coarsely chopped

3 large tomatoes, coarsely chopped

2/3 cup red onion, coarsely chopped

1/3 cup balsamic vinegar

1/2 tbsp white sugar

3 tablespoons extra virgin olive oil

Salt and pepper, to taste

Fresh basil or mint leaves, for garnish (optional)

Directions

In a large bowl with a lid, combine all ingredients. Cover, and shake to mix.

Season with salt and pepper.

RADICCHIO, TOMATO AND CRESS SALAD

Ingredients

60 g (1 ½ cups) shredded radicchio

120 g (3 cups) shredded Romaine

10 cherry tomatoes (170 g), halved

2 large stalks celery (130 g), sliced

60 g (2 oz) unpeeled cucumber, diced

40 g (1.4 oz) garden cress, trimmed

2 tsp extra virgin olive oil

2 tsp vinegar

Directions

Place the radicchio, romaine, cherry tomatoes, celery and cucumber in a large bowl. Toss well.

Add the olive oil and vinegar to the salad mix and toss again lightly.

Serve immediately.

Wholesome Winter Pea and Watercress Soup (Dairy-Free

Ingredients

1 large onion

1 garlic clove

6 cups vegetable or chicken stock

1 zucchini

30 oz frozen peas

3 oz watercress

Salt and pepper, to taste

Directions

Peel and crush the garlic and set aside. Leaving crushed or minced garlic for at least 5-10 minutes after crushing helps maximize its health-protective effects.

While health-promoting compounds are forming in crushed garlic, wash and trim the zucchini, and cut it into chunks.

Peel and chop the onion, and sweat it, together with the minced garlic, in 2-3 tablespoons of chicken or vegetable stock in a stock pot.

Add the zucchini chunks and pour in the rest of the stock. Bring to a boil and simmer for until the zucchini chunks are just cooked, about 10 minutes.

Add the frozen peas and simmer for 3 minutes. Add the watercress and simmer for another minute.

Remove from the heat and let cool for a few minutes. Process with a hand-held blender until smooth. Season with salt.

CHICKEN SOUP WITH RICE AND BROCCOLI

Ingredients

4 cups fat-free, low-sodium chicken broth

1 small onion, chopped

1 1/2 cups broccoli florets

2 small ribs organic celery, diced

2 small carrots, sliced

1/2 cup short grain brown rice, washed

2 cups cooked, skinless chicken, diced

Directions

Soak rice in cold water from 15 minutes to one hour. This will reduce cooking time.

Bring broth to a boil in a large saucepan. Add presoaked rice and vegetables. Reduce heat to low, cover and simmer, stirring occasionally, until rice is tender.

Add cooked chicken and simmer for 3-4 minutes.

Did you know?

While both broccoli stem and florets are edible, the broccoli florets are generally thought to be healthier as they provide more vitamins and cancer-fighting substances than the stem.

TANGY TOMATO SOUP WITH BASIL

Ingredients

3 large garlic cloves

3 oz shallots, peeled sliced

1 Tbsp olive oil

1 (14 1/2-ounce) can stewed tomatoes, undrained

1 1/2 cups chicken broth

1/2 tsp apple cider vinegar

1/4 tsp salt

Dash of freshly ground red pepper

2 tbsp fresh basil, chopped

Directions

Peel and crush garlic and set aside. Leaving crushed or minced garlic for at least 5-10 minutes after crushing helps maximize its health-protective effects.

While health-promoting compounds are forming in crushed garlic, combine shallots, tomatoes, chicken broth, and apple cider vinegar in a blender or food processor and process until smooth.

Heat olive oil in a large nonstick saucepan over medium heat. Add garlic and cook about 30 seconds, stirring constantly.

Add tomato mixture, and bring to a boil. Turn off heat and stir in basil. Serve hot

Broccoli and Barley Soup

Ingredients

1/4 cup yellow onion, chopped

1 small carrot, peeled and diced

1 rib organic celery, finely chopped

1 tbsp extra virgin olive oil

4 cups small, organic broccoli florets

1/2 cup pearled barley, cooked

5 cups vegetable broth

1 can (14 1/2 oz) stewed tomatoes

4 cloves garlic, minced

1/4 tsp dried marjoram

1 tsp thyme

Salt and pepper, to taste

Directions

In a stock pot, cook onion in olive oil over medium heat for 4-5 minutes until soft.

Add vegetable broth and bring to a boil. Reduce to a simmer and add celery and carrots along with broccoli florets. Cover and let simmer until carrots and broccoli florets are tender.

Add cooked barley, canned tomatoes, garlic, marjoram, and thyme. Let simmer another minute or two.

Season with salt and pepper. Serve warm.

NOURISHING NETTLE SOUP

Ingredients

6 oz young nettle tips

4 oz fresh spinach

2 tbsp olive oil

2 shallots, chopped

2 cups water

2 cups skimmed organic milk

3 tbsp flour

Dash of ground white pepper

Dash of ground nutmeg

Salt to taste

Yoghurt with probiotic bacteria, for garnish

Directions

Wash nettle and spinach thoroughly. Drain and chop coarsely.

Heat olive oil and sauté onion in a large saucepan until golden brown.

Stir-Fried Asparagus with Quinoa Noodles

Ingredients

2 bundles asparagus, washed, trimmed, and cut into bite-size pieces

1 tbsp olive oil

3 tsp fresh ginger, minced

2 garlic cloves, slivered

1 tbsp soy sauce

1/2 tbsp sugar

3 1/2 tbsp vegetable stock

12 oz dried quinoa noodles

Directions

Heat oil in a wok and stir-fry ginger and garlic for a minute or two, then add asparagus.

Combine soy sauce, sugar, and stock in a small bowl and pour over asparagus. Simmer until asparagus is tender, about 3-5 minutes.

Cook noodles according to package directions and serve with stir-fried asparagus.

ACE SALAD

Ingredients

6 organic carrots, thinly sliced

1 fennel bulb, thinly sliced

1 cucumber, thinly sliced

1 cup fresh parsley, chopped

4 Tbsp freshly squeezed lemon juice

2 Tbsp extra virgin olive oil

Sea salt

Freshly ground black pepper

Directions

Combine carrots, fennel, cucumber, and parsley in a large bowl.

Mix lemon juice, olive oil, salt, and pepper in a container with a securable lid. Tighten lid and shake.

Pour dressing over salad and toss gently.

Salmon Salad

Ingredients

2 large fillets (9 oz) wild salmon, either poached or grilled and chilled in the fridge until cool

1 cup cherry tomatoes, halved

2 red onions, sliced

1 tbsp capers

1 tablespoon fresh dill, finely chopped

1 tbsp balsamic vinegar

1 tbsp olive oil

1/4 tsp pepper, freshly ground

Pinch of salt

Directions

When salmon is cool, remove skin and bones. Break into chunks and add to a bowl.

Add tomatoes, red onion, and capers. Toss.

Mix vinegar, olive oil, and dill in a small bowl and add pour over salmon chunks. Toss again.

Add salt and pepper to taste. Refrigerate for at least 30 minutes before serving

BEET AND CARROT SOUP

Ingredients

3 medium beets, peeled and diced

1 tbsp olive oil

1 cup onion, chopped

1 pound carrots, diced

1 tbsp fresh ginger, minced

1 garlic clove, minced

6 cups vegetable stock

Directions

Heat oil in a large saucepan over medium heat. Sauté onion until golden brown. Add ginger and garlic and cook for 2 minutes, stirring frequently.

Add beets, carrots, and stock. Reduce heat to low and simmer covered until beets and carrots are tender, about 25 minutes.

In a food processor, purée soup in batches. Taste soup and adjust seasonings.

Serve hot or cold, garnished with cilantro leaves.

Arugula, Avocado and Tomato Salad

Ingredients

3 cups young arugula leaves, rinsed

2 cups cherry tomatoes, halved

1/4 cup sun-dried tomatoes, chopped

2 tablespoons extra virgin olive oil

1 tablespoon balsamic vinegar

2 small avocados, peeled, pitted and sliced

Directions

In a large plastic bowl with a lid, combine arugula, cherry tomatoes, sun-dried tomatoes, olive oil, and vinegar. Toss well.

Divide onto plates, and top each serving with slices of avocado.

BEET AND CARROT SALAD WITH GINGER

Ingredients

1/2 cup raw beets, peeled and grated

1/2 cup organic carrots, grated

2 tbsp apple juice

1 tbsp extra-virgin olive oil

1/2 tsp fresh ginger, minced

1/8 tsp sea salt

Directions

Combine grated beets and carrots in a small bowl.

Mix apple juice, olive oil, ginger, and salt in a separate bowl and drizzle over salad mixture. Toss gently. Enjoy!

Did you know?

Beta-carotene, found in many orange vegetables such as carrots, is a fat-soluble vitamin, which means that it has to be consumed together with a little bit of fat in order for it to be absorbed and utilized by the body. Therefore, the essential fatty acids provided by the olive oil in this recipe are an ideal accompaniment for carrots.

Carrot and Avocado Salad

Ingredients

1 large avocado, peeled, pitted and diced

4 medium carrots, peeled and grated

Dash of balsamic vinegar

Sunflower seeds, to taste

Salt and freshly ground pepper, to taste

Directions

Combine avocado and grated carrots in a medium salad bowl. Sprinkle with sunflower seeds, salt, pepper, and balsamic vinegar.

Cover and refrigerate for at least 20 minutes before serving.

ANTI-CERVICAL CANCER BREAKFAST RECIPES

Buckwheat Pancakes with Papaya Purée

Ingredients

1 cup buckwheat flour

1 Tbsp brown sugar

2 Tbsp potato starch

1/2 tsp salt

1 tsp baking powder

1 cup rice milk

2 Tbsp canola oil

Vegetable cooking spray, for frying

2 papayas, peeled, seeded and diced

Brown rice syrup, to serve

Directions

Combine dry ingredients in a medium bowl. Add rice milk

and canola oil, and whisk until well combined. If batter seems very thick, you may want add a little extra rice milk or water.

Preheat a large nonstick skillet over medium heat. Spray with vegetable cooking spray.

With a ladle, pour batter to the size you prefer. Even out batter on skillet with back of a spoon. Cook pancake on medium high heat for a few minutes until bubbles appear. Flip over and continue frying until cooked (a properly cooked pancake appears dense and not sticky when cut in the middle).

Repeat previous step until batter is gone.

Purée diced papaya in a food processor. Ladle into a serving bowl.

Serve pancakes with papaya purée and brown rice syrup.

ORIGINAL BIRCHER MUESLI

Ingredients

1 tbsp rolled oats

3 tbsp water

1 tbsp sweetened condensed milk

2 tsp lemon juice

1-2 apples (including skin)

1 tbsp hazelnuts or almonds, ground

Directions

Combine oats and water and refrigerate overnight. Soaking improves the nutritional value of oats as it allows enzymes to break down and neutralize phytic acid, a compound that can block the absorption of many minerals in the intestines.

Grate apples. Add them, together with sweetened condensed milk and lemon juice, to soaked oats. Stir well.

Sprinkle with almonds or hazelnuts and serve.

Did you know?

Soaking improves the nutritional value of oats as it allows enzymes to break down and neutralize phytic acid, a compound that can block the absorption of many minerals in the intestines.

Dairy-Free Blueberry Muesli

Ingredients

1 1/2 cups rolled oats

1/2 cup walnuts, chopped

1/2 cup dried apples, chopped

2 tsp ground cinnamon

2 cups blueberries (preferably wild)

3 tbsp brown sugar

Apple juice, to serve

Directions

Preheat oven to 325°F (160°C, gas 3).

Mix oats, sugar, and cinnamon in a bowl. Spread mixture evenly onto a non-stick baking tray.

Toast oat mixture in preheated oven for about 10 minutes, stirring occasionally. Watch mixture very closely when toasting as it can burn very easily.

Antioxidant Muffins

Ingredients

1 cup whole wheat flour

1/3 cup brown sugar

1/2 tsp baking powder

1/3 cup pecans, chopped

1/4 tsp salt

1 cup blueberries

1/4 cup almond milk

1 large egg

Directions

Preheat oven to 350°F (175°C, gas 4).

Combine flour, sugar, baking powder, pecans, and salt. In a separate bowl, lightly beat egg and almond milk. Combine dry and wet ingredients.

Pour batter into paper muffin cups. Bake for 30-40 minutes, then transfer muffins to a cooling rack. Serve warm.

CARROT MUFFINS

Ingredients

1 egg

1 cup rice milk

4 tbsp canola oil

2 cups quinoa flour or other gluten-free flour

1 tsp guar gum

1 tbsp flaxseed meal

3 1/2 tsp gluten-free baking powder

1/2 tsp salt

1 tsp cinnamon

1/4 cup brown sugar

1 cup organic carrots, grated

1/4 cup raisins

Directions

Preheat oven to 400 degrees F (200 degrees C, gas mark 6)

Beat together egg, rice milk, and canola oil. Combine dry ingredients in a separate bowl.

Add liquid ingredients to dry ingredients and mix until just blended (do not over-mix). Fold in grated carrots and raisins.

Fill 12 paper muffin cups with batter (about two thirds full). Bake for 20 minutes.

CERVICAL CANCER FIGHTING SOUP RECIPES

Red Cabbage Soup with Black Lentils

Ingredients

½ cup (96 g) black lentils

2 Tbsp (30 ml) olive oil

2 cloves (6 g) garlic

1 small onion (70 g)

½ red cabbage (420 g), shredded

2 ½ US cups (591 ml) low-sodium vegetable stock

½ broccoli (304 g), coarsely chopped

10 sprigs (5 g) fresh thyme, chopped

Directions

Prepare and cook the lentils according to the instructions on the package. While the lentils are cooking, chop the garlic and onions, and let them sit for 15 minutes to allow them to produce allicin, a health promoting compound that is formed when Allium vegetables such as garlic and onions are chopped.

Heat the olive oil in a large pan and add the garlic, onion, and red cabbage. Cook for a few minutes.

Add the vegetable stock and bring to a boil, then add the broccoli. Reduce heat, and simmer until the broccoli is tender. This generally takes about 8-10 minutes. Turn off the heat and stir in the cooked lentils. Add the thyme and serve immediately.

Apple and Onion Soup

Ingredients

1 Tbsp canola oil

2 medium yellow onions, sliced

1 small leek, chopped

1/2 Tbsp fresh rosemary, chopped

1/2 Tbsp fresh thyme

3 organic apples, cut into small dices

6 cups fat-free, low-sodium vegetable broth

Directions

Heat the oil in a medium saucepan over medium heat. Add the onions and sauté until golden.

Pour in the broth and bring to the boil over medium-high

heat. Add the apples, and reduce the heat to medium-low. Simmer for 10 minutes.

Nutritional Information

Nutrition facts for this Apple and Onion Soup are provided per 100 grams, per recipe (2321 grams), and per portion (387 grams) in the table below. The Percent Daily Values are provided in brackets.

GRANDMA'S CHICKEN SOUP

Ingredients

4 cups fat-free, low-sodium chicken broth

1 onion, chopped

3/4 cup sweet potato, diced

3/4 cup turnip, diced

2 ribs organic celery, diced

2 carrots, sliced

1/2 cup fresh parsley, chopped

2 cups skinless, organic chicken, cooked and diced

Directions

Bring broth to a boil in a large saucepan, and add vege-tables. Reduce heat to low, cover and simmer, until vege-tables are tender.

Add cooked chicken and simmer for 3-4 minutes.

Wholesome Winter Pea and Watercress Soup (Dairy-Free)

Ingredients

1 large onion

1 garlic clove

6 cups vegetable or chicken stock

1 zucchini

30 oz frozen peas

3 oz watercress

Salt and pepper, to taste

Directions

Peel and crush the garlic and set aside. Leaving crushed or minced garlic for at least 5-10 minutes after crushing helps maximize its health-protective effects.

While health-promoting compounds are forming in crushed garlic, wash and trim the zucchini, and cut it into chunks.

Peel and chop the onion, and sweat it, together with the minced garlic, in 2-3 tablespoons of chicken or vegetable stock in a stock pot.

Add the zucchini chunks and pour in the rest of the stock. Bring to a boil and simmer for until the zucchini chunks are just cooked, about 10 minutes.

Add the frozen peas and simmer for 3 minutes. Add the watercress and simmer for another minute.

Remove from the heat and let cool for a few minutes. Process with a hand-held blender until smooth. Season with salt.

NOURISHING NETTLE SOUP

Ingredients

6 oz young nettle tips

4 oz fresh spinach

2 tbsp olive oil

2 shallots, chopped

2 cups water

2 cups skimmed organic milk

3 tbsp flour

Dash of ground white pepper

Dash of ground nutmeg

Salt to taste

Yoghurt with probiotic bacteria, for garnish

Directions

Wash nettle and spinach thoroughly. Drain and chop coarsely.

Heat olive oil and sauté onion in a large saucepan until golden brown.

Add water, nettle, and spinach, and bring to a boil. Cook until nettle and spinach are tender. Blend with a hand held blender until smooth.

Whisk cold milk and flour together in a small bowl. Pour into saucepan and whisk to blend thoroughly.

Bring to a boil and simmer for a few minutes, until thickened. Season with salt, white pepper, and nutmeg. Remove from heat.

Pour soup into serving bowls and garnish with a swirl of yoghurt. Serve.

Note: As nettles are rich in nitrates, they should not be consumed by young children, people with gout, or other people with a condition that requires a low-nitrate diet.

Tangy Tomato Soup with Basil

Ingredients

3 large garlic cloves

3 oz shallots, peeled sliced

1 Tbsp olive oil

1 (14 1/2-ounce) can stewed tomatoes, undrained

1 1/2 cups chicken broth

1/2 tsp apple cider vinegar

1/4 tsp salt

Dash of freshly ground red pepper

2 tbsp fresh basil, chopped

Directions

Peel and crush garlic and set aside. Leaving crushed or minced garlic for at least 5-10 minutes after crushing helps maximize its health-protective effects.

While health-promoting compounds are forming in crushed garlic, combine shallots, tomatoes, chicken broth, and apple cider vinegar in a blender or food processor and process until smooth.

Heat olive oil in a large nonstick saucepan over medium heat. Add garlic and cook about 30 seconds, stirring constantly.

Add tomato mixture, and bring to a boil. Turn off heat and stir in basil. Serve hot

Chicken Soup with Rice and Broccoli

Ingredients

4 cups fat-free, low-sodium chicken broth

1 small onion, chopped

1 1/2 cups broccoli florets

2 small ribs organic celery, diced

2 small carrots, sliced

1/2 cup short grain brown rice, washed

2 cups cooked, skinless chicken, diced

Directions

Soak rice in cold water from 15 minutes to one hour. This will reduce cooking time.

Bring broth to a boil in a large saucepan. Add presoaked rice and vegetables. Reduce heat to low, cover and simmer, stirring occasionally, until rice is tender.

Add cooked chicken and simmer for 3-4 minutes.

BROCCOLI AND BARLEY SOUP

Ingredients

1/4 cup yellow onion, chopped

1 small carrot, peeled and diced

1 rib organic celery, finely chopped

1 tbsp extra virgin olive oil

4 cups small, organic broccoli florets

1/2 cup pearled barley, cooked

5 cups vegetable broth

1 can (14 1/2 oz) stewed tomatoes

4 cloves garlic, minced

1/4 tsp dried marjoram

1 tsp thyme

Salt and pepper, to taste

Directions

In a stock pot, cook onion in olive oil over medium heat

for 4-5 minutes until soft.

Add vegetable broth and bring to a boil. Reduce to a simmer and add celery and carrots along with broccoli florets. Cover and let simmer until carrots and broccoli florets are tender.

Add cooked barley, canned tomatoes, garlic, marjoram, and thyme. Let simmer another minute or two.

Season with salt and pepper. Serve warm.

BEET AND CARROT SOUP

Ingredients

3 medium beets, peeled and diced

1 tbsp olive oil

1 cup onion, chopped

1 pound carrots, diced

1 tbsp fresh ginger, minced

1 garlic clove, minced

6 cups vegetable stock

Directions

Heat oil in a large saucepan over medium heat. Sauté onion until golden brown. Add ginger and garlic and cook for 2 minutes, stirring frequently.

Add beets, carrots, and stock. Reduce heat to low and simmer covered until beets and carrots are tender, about 25 minutes.

In a food processor, purée soup in batches. Taste soup and adjust seasonings.

Serve hot or cold, garnished with cilantro leaves.

CERVICAL CANCER FIGHTING SMOOTHIES AND OTHER DRINKS (RECIPES)

Grape Juice and Raspberry Smoothie

Ingredients

1/2 cup raspberries, rinsed

1 banana, sliced (Day 1*)

1 ½ cups red grape juice

2 Tbsp sunflower seeds

1 tsp turmeric powder

½ cup crushed ice

Directions

Place the raspberries, banana, red grape juice, sunflower seeds, turmeric powder, and crushed ice in a blender (note: if you're using a high-powered blender that can handle whole ice cubes, you can also use eight ice cubes instead of crushed ice if you like).

Secure the lid and blend until smooth.

Pour into glasses and enjoy immediately.

GREEN TEA MANGO BLAST

Ingredients

2 cups mango, peeled and chopped

1 cup green tea made from loose leaves

1 Tbsp honey

1/2 inch piece fresh ginger, peeled and finely chopped

1 cup crushed ice

Directions

Combine all ingredients in a blender or food processor and process until smooth.

Garnish as desired, and serve with eco-straws made of stainless steel, bamboo, or tough borosilicate glass.

Blood Orange and Raspberry Smoothie

Ingredients

¾ cup blood orange juice

1 ½ cups (185 g) raspberries

2 teaspoons flaxseed oil

½ cup crushed ice

Fresh mint, for garnish

Directions

Blend the blood orange juice, raspberries, and flaxseed oil in a blender or food processor until smooth.

Add the crushed ice and mix again.

Pour into into small glasses and garnish with fresh mint. Serve with quirky eco-straws made of stainless steel, glass, or bamboo.

SCANDINAVIAN BLUEBERRY SOUP

Ingredients

4 cups blueberries

2 cup water

1/2 cup sugar

4 tbsp potato starch

Directions

Place blueberries, sugar, and water into a saucepan and bring to a boil.

Mix potato starch with a few drops of cold water and stir into blueberry mixture. Continue stirring over low heat until soup thickens.

Pour into a serving dish and serve immediately. Alternatively, you can sprinkle soup with a bit of sugar, cool it in the fridge, and serve chilled.

Did you know?

To fully benefit from the antioxidant powers of blueberries, it is best to eat blueberry dishes without dairy. In a recent study, volunteers were given 200 grams (7 ounces) of blueberries with either 200 ml (0.8 cups) of water or 200 ml milk. Those who consumed blueberries with water had a significant increase in their plasma antioxidant capacity. Interestingly, this effect was not found in those volunteers who ingested blueberries with milk. The study authors believe that the ability of milk to impair the anti-oxidant powers of blueberries may be a result of blueberries' natural affinity for milk protein.

SUPERFOOD SMOOTHIE FOR CANCER AND CVD PREVENTION

Ingredients

1 ½ cups frozen organic strawberries

1 tsp chia seeds (buy chia seeds here)

1 small organic banana

1 cup red grapes

1 ¼ cup unsweetened cranberry juice

Directions

Rinse the frozen strawberries under cold running water, and let them thaw for 15 minutes. Prepare the chia seeds by soaking them in cold water for 15 minutes.

While your strawberries are thawing and your chia seeds are soaking up water, peel banana and rinse the grapes.

Add the thawed strawberries, soaked chia seeds, banana, grapes and cranberry juice to a large-capacity blender, secure the lid, and process until nice and smooth.

Pour into glasses, garnish as desired, and serve immediately.

CATECHIN-RICH ICE TEA

Ingredients

2 cups water

2 1/2 tsp loose green tea leaves

(loose leaves release more catechins than tea bags)

3 Tbsp freshly pressed organic lemon juice

Directions

Boil the water. Place green tea leaves in tea pot and pour boiling water into the pot. Let steep five minutes.

Strain the tea and add lemon juice (lemon juice is rich in vitamin C which helps make the catechins contained in green tea more available to the body).

Refrigerate until completely chilled before serving.

Serve with eco-friendly straws made of tough borosilicate glass, stainless steel, or bamboo.

Raspberry Blueberry Smoothie

Ingredients

1 cup fresh raspberries

1 cup wild blueberries

3/4 cup rice milk

3/4 cup crushed ice

1 Tbsp flaxseed, freshly ground

Directions

Combine all ingredients in a blender or food processor and process until smooth.

Garnish as desired, and serve with eco-straws which are good both for you and the environment.

CONCLUSION

A plan for the diagnosis and treatment of cancer is a key component of any overall cancer control plan. Its main goal is to cure cancer patients or prolong their life considerably, ensuring a good quality of life. In order for a diagnosis and treatment programme to be effective, it must never be developed in isolation. It needs to be linked to an early detection programme so that cases are detected at an early stage, when treatment is more effective and there is a greater chance of cure. It also needs to be integrated with a palliative care programme, so that patients with advanced cancers, who can no longer benefit from treatment, will get adequate relief from their physical, psychosocial and spiritual suffering. Furthermore, programmes should include a awareness-raising component, to educate patients, family and community members about the cancer risk factors and the need for taking preventive measures to avoid developing cancer.

Where resources are limited, diagnosis and treatment services should initially target all patients presenting with curable cancers, such as breast, cervical and oral cancers that can be detected early. They could also include childhood acute lymphatic leukaemia, which has a high potential for cure although it cannot be detected early. Above all, services need to be provided in an equitable and sustainable manner. As and when more resources become available, the programme can be extended to include

other curable cancers as well as cancers for which treatment can prolong survival considerably.